I Love To Jump Rope:

The Jump Roping Handbook For Better Fitness And Health

Written By
Angela Bentley-Henry, M.Ed.

Contents

Chapter 1: I Love to Jump Rope 1

Chapter 2: The Benefits 5

Chapter 3: The Basics 11

Chapter 4: Accessories 15

Chapter 5: The Jump Rope Tricks 18

Chapter 6: Time to Train 31

Chapter 7: The Workouts 43

Chapter 8: The Acceleration Process 67

Chapter 9: No Pain, No Setbacks 74

Chapter 10: "Just In Case" 77

About the Author 90

Special Thanks 92

Reference 94

This book is dedicated to my daughters, Abriana and Aleah. Thanks for jumping with Mommy ☺.

DISCLAIMER

I am not a doctor, physician, or healthcare provider. I cannot heal, treat, or cure you of any health-related illnesses. You understand that this book is not intended as a substitute for consultation with a licensed healthcare practitioner, such as your physician. Before you begin any healthcare program (fitness or nutrition program), or change your lifestyle in anyway, you should consult your physician or other licensed healthcare practitioner to ensure that you are in good health and that the examples and information contained in this book will not harm you. The use of any information provided in this book is solely at your own risk.

Chapter 1

I Love to Jump Rope

I want to start off by saying, I LOVE TO JUMP ROPE. Absolutely, without question, love it. Now that that is established, I have a few questions to ask you:

Why did you decide to pick up this jump rope handbook?

Are you trying to lose weight? Are you currently battling a lifestyle or chronic disease? Are you trying to eliminate body fat? Are you working to improve your athletic ability? Are you looking to make your workouts more interesting?

If you answered yes to any of those questions, then you are in the right place! I have found throughout my health and fitness journey that when the process begins to be enjoyable, it is easier to stay consistent. The consistency is what makes fitness a lifestyle versus a quick fix. When you approach fitness and health with this mindset, results tend to follow.

My desire to meet my health and fitness goals is what led me to the jump rope.

My journey to pursuing a lifelong healthy lifestyle began in 2015. I would like to say that I woke up one day and "chose" to make health and fitness a priority, but that wouldn't be the full truth. The full truth is that a health scare pushed me into health and fitness. I had no choice but to change my lifestyle.

In October 2015, I went for my annual physical and blood work, and was deemed overweight and diagnosed with prediabetes. My physician offered me no real solutions. Basically, I was told that as the diabetes progressed, I would be given the appropriate medication. In terms of nutrition and fitness, the only direction given was to "eat healthy and exercise". Not much detail included in that advice, right?

For me, the prediabetes diagnosis was a major wake-up call and scary. You see, just a few months earlier, June 2015, my grandmother had passed away after a 20-year battle with diabetes. Unfortunately, I had seen firsthand how diabetes could destroy a person's quality of life, and I did not want that for myself or for my family.

After feeling down and defeated, I picked myself up and made up my mind that there would be no diabetes progression, and I would lose the unnecessary weight. I decided that the vague medical advice I was given coupled with the looming prescriptions would not be my future.

The process of becoming the "healthier and fit" version of myself began with lots of research. I earned several certifications, read nutrition and fitness related books and watched countless plant-based nutrition documentaries, all in an attempt to find solutions.

Using this combination of information, I changed my nutritional habits and focused on my overall health and fitness. My new-found pursuit led me to the jump rope, a plant-dominated diet, and a different outlook on healthy living.

When I first started jumping (again), I grabbed an old jump rope buried deep in my garage and just jumped. I had not jumped in years; I mean, not for real. I knew how to jump "playground style" but had never actually studied the mechanics of jumping rope as an adult. Being who I am, I became obsessed with learning everything there was to learn about jumping rope and was eager to apply the information.

I figured some accountability would be a fun way to try out what I was learning as I was learning it. I came across an 100-jump per day challenge on Instagram that was being hosted by a social media influencer I followed, Bernadette Henry (no relation), and decided to join. She is better known on social media as "Make it Fun NYC". She was/is an amazing jumper, and I was eager to join the challenge to reach my goals.

After the 100-jump challenge, I was hooked more than ever! I was even more in love with jumping rope. I was determined to use jumping rope to not only reach my health and fitness goals, but I also wanted to be GREAT AT JUMPING.

From that point forward, my weekly schedule consisted of jumping rope, working out, and trying to learn new jump rope tricks. I could tell the consistency was paying off. I saw my physique improving, the weight was dropping, and I was having so much fun doing it.

By the time January 2016 rolled around, I was 15 pounds lighter, was able to do a ton of new jump rope tricks, my body was leaner all over, and according to my blood work, I was no longer prediabetic! I felt amazing.

I couldn't wait to share what I had learned and what I love with the world. I started sharing health and fitness related information on social media, earned my fitness trainer license, weight management specialist certification, plant-based cooking certification, punk rope jump rope instructor certification, and began hosting my own jump rope workout classes locally.

PUNK ROPE JUMP ROPE CLASSES

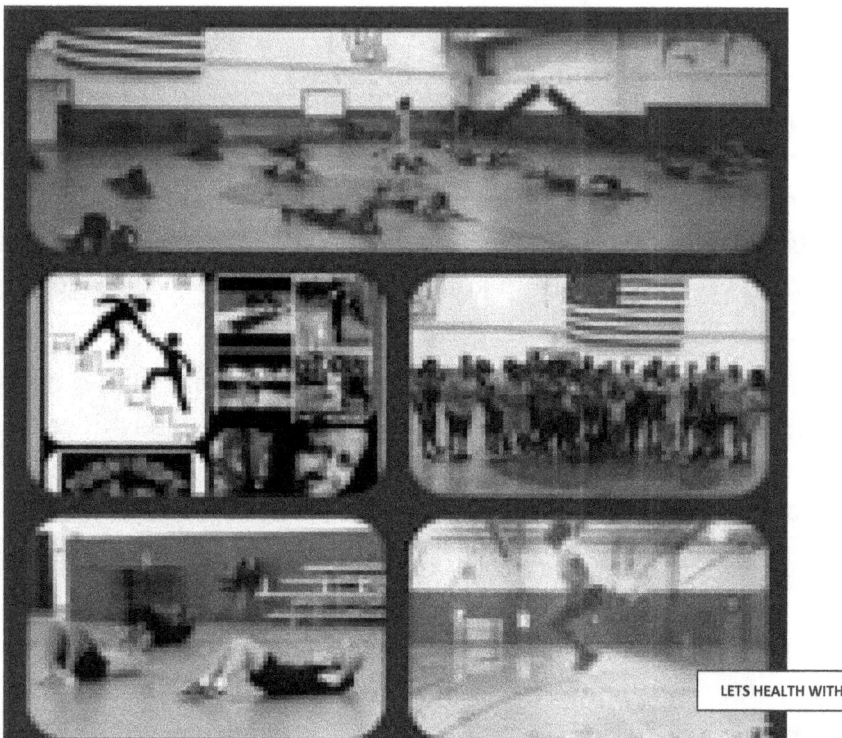

Participants were having so much fun and reaching their fitness goals. It was wonderful.

Although I'm not currently hosting any jump rope courses, being able to offer challenges from time to time and writing this handbook is my way of sharing "cheat codes", and hopefully inspiring others to love jumping rope as well.

Enjoy the journey you are about to embark on. I am sure you will share in my excitement and love of jumping rope by the end of this experience!

CHAPTER 2

THE BENEFITS

If you have ever picked up a jump rope and started jumping for the first time (or for the first time in a long time), you usually start smiling (because it is fun), but then after a few jumps you begin to think to yourself that this isn't as easy as you thought it would be. Your heart begins to speed up. Your arms, core, and, of course, lower body begin to feel "it" after a while. That's when it hits you—you are getting a great full body workout right now.

Not only will you improve your cardiovascular system (cardio), but because of the strength and explosiveness required to jump repeatedly, you will not have to worry about losing muscle while training.

Throughout my weight loss and fitness journey, which unfortunately has not always been perfect nor linear, jumping rope has allowed me to get the best results in the shortest amount of time. I know I have already shared with you why "I LOVE TO JUMP ROPE", but the appreciation goes deeper than just my personal testimony. I also love to jump rope because of the numerous benefits.

These benefits really stick out:
1. Jump ropes are portable and inexpensive.

2. Jumping rope burns a lot of calories in a short amount of time.
3. Jumping rope may improve a person's cardiovascular endurance.
4. Jumping rope may improve muscular endurance.
5. Jumping rope may improve body composition.
6. Jumping rope may improve coordination and other skill related components of physical fitness.
7. Jumping rope is a mood enhancing activity.
8. Jumping rope is convenient.

Benefit #1

Jump ropes are *inexpensive and very portable*. A typical jump rope can be purchased for around 10 bucks. They fit nicely in a bag and are lightweight enough to pack up and take anywhere.

Benefit #2

Jumping rope tends to *burn a lot of calories in a short amount of time*. I am often asked, "How many calories will I burn in a jump rope workout?" The answer is not as simple as most other forms of exercise. There are a few factors to consider, like the weight of the person jumping, the intensity level (jumping tempo), type of jump rope tricks, and the duration of the jump rope session. The more someone weighs and how intensely they jump will affect the calories they can potentially burn while jumping rope.

According to

https://caloriesburnedhq.com/calories-burned-jumping-rope/, jumping rope can burn 15 to 20 calories per minute. Also, according to

https://caloriesburnedhq.com/calories-burned-jumping-rope/, the average person could burn 200 to 300 calories in a 15-minute jump rope session.

Benefit #3

Jumping rope improves many of the health-related components of physical fitness. The 5 health related components are: cardiovascular endurance, muscular strength, muscular endurance, flexibility, and body composition.

Cardiovascular endurance is the measure of how long and effectively one's heart and lungs can "work". Jumping rope is a *great cardiovascular (heart and lung health) improving activity*. Although there are other forms of cardiovascular activities that are great as well, such as running, cycling, or swimming, jumping rope tends to accelerate the heart rate more quickly and therefore allows the body to make improvements in a short amount of time.

Jumping rope consistently may improve a person's overall heart health and the way the heart and the lungs work together to provide oxygen to the rest of the body. Having strong heart health may reduce a person's chances of heart disease or stroke.

A study published in *The Research Quarterly*, a journal of the American Association for Health, Physical Education and Research, titled "Comparison of Rope Skipping and Jogging as Methods of Improving Cardiovascular Efficiency of College Men", conducted a 6-week study of 92 students. It was concluded that jumping rope for 10 minutes will improve cardiovascular efficiency just as much as jogging for 30 minutes would (as measured by the Harvard step test) (Baker J.A. 1968). Wow, right?! So, in addition to being amazing for the cardiovascular system, jumping rope is also very time efficient.

Benefit #4

While engaging several major muscles of the body, jumping rope may also *enhance a person's muscular endurance*. As stated before, muscular endurance is a component of physical fitness, which is a measure of how long a particular muscle can be used before it tires out. For example, let's say we have a person who can lift 200 pounds on the bench press, and they can lift that amount of weight, 15 or more times, before eventually tiring out. The number of repetitions or length of time they are able to sustain that weight would be a measure of their endurance for their pectoralis (chest) muscle (triceps and other muscles engaged) while completing a bench press.

When jumping rope, there are several major muscles that are being "worked until they tire", seeing as a person is responsible for lifting their body weight off the ground repeatedly.

The major muscles that are used while jumping rope are the hamstrings, glutes, quadriceps, and calves, but the beauty of jumping rope is it also engages the deltoids, biceps, triceps, abdominals, and back muscles. This is why jumping rope is considered a full body exercise.

Benefit #5

Body composition is a percentage that represents the amount of body fat, bones, and muscle mass in a person's body. The higher the number (percentage), the more body fat present in a person's body. Although this percentage is helpful in identifying risk, it shouldn't be relied on solely as an assessment of a person's health.

Between muscular endurance and the major muscles that are engaged during jumping rope, jumping rope maybe *an excellent way to improve a person's body composition*. Jumping rope, combined with good nutrition, may help the body become leaner overall.

There are numerous body composition and body mass index calculators online if you want to know what your current percentage is.

Benefit #6

The skill-related components of physical fitness are agility, speed, power, balance, coordination, and reaction time. Jumping rope tends to improve all of the skill-related components.

Athletes and fitness enthusiasts often include jumping rope as a part of their training plans. Jumping rope helps take their sports specific skills to another level, and the skills required to be a "great jumper" are transferable to other types of fitness activities.

Arguably, *one of the biggest skills that is improved upon from jumping rope is coordination.* Coordination is the body's ability to use body parts and senses together during activity. For example, when speaking of coordination, you often hear of hand eye coordination and/or foot eye coordination. This is the coordination of hand movement based on what the eyes see, and equally, foot movement based on what the eyes see. Jumping rope will help pretty much any activity or sport that you have to be able to change direction quickly, or where reaction time and balance are key, (for example, basketball and boxing).

The jump rope is very unforgiving for a lack of coordination. The jump rope forces you to improve your coordination by giving you immediate feedback. You will either hit yourself with the rope if coordination, reaction time, and balance are still developing or successfully jump over the rope if your coordination has progressed.

Benefit #7

Jumping rope is a *mood enhancer*. I like to call it "therapy". Jumping rope releases, as people like to call them, feel-good endorphins. These endorphins are neurotransmitters produced by the brain during activity.

These endorphins help relieve anxiety, stress, depression, and leave the exerciser with a lingering sense of calmness and happiness. Yes, this is experienced during other types of exercise, but we are discussing the jump rope right now.

Benefit #8 Convenient

The jump rope is so portable and doesn't require a lot of space to jump that it *makes jumping rope very convenient.* You can jump rope at home, on vacation, at work, or wherever. You no longer need a gym membership to be fit. You also do not need anyone's assistance to jump rope. It is an individual job activity.

Chapter 3

The Basics

Embarking on a new fitness journey can be intimidating. Restarting a fitness journey can be just as intimidating. What tends to lessen the intimidation and help the startup, or the "start back", to be more comfortable is knowing the fitness activity vocabulary and knowing the basic tips for success of the fitness activity. This chapter will focus on many of the basic essentials to the jump rope and the skill of jump roping.

What you need to get started
1. A jump rope
2. A positive attitude

Common types of jump ropes
1. PVC rope – Very durable. Can be used indoors or outdoors. Does not kink or tangle. I recommend it for beginners.
2. Nylon Rope – Tough rope. Can handle tough concrete. Good for kids and beginners. Typically has a slower rotation, which is helpful when first beginning to jump.

What else you need to get started
1. A good pair of athletic shoes
2. An open mind

Sizing your jump rope

1. Hold your jump rope in both hands (as if you were going to start jumping).
2. Place your dominate foot on the center of the rope.
3. Hold the handles together towards your shoulder area. The length should fall between your shoulders and your armpit.
4. The handles should be closer to the armpit if you consider yourself an intermediate to advanced jumper.
5. The handles should be closer to your shoulders if you consider yourself a beginner.

Where to jump rope

1. Indoor gym floor
2. Fitness workout room
3. On a jumping mat (see "The Accessories" chapter)

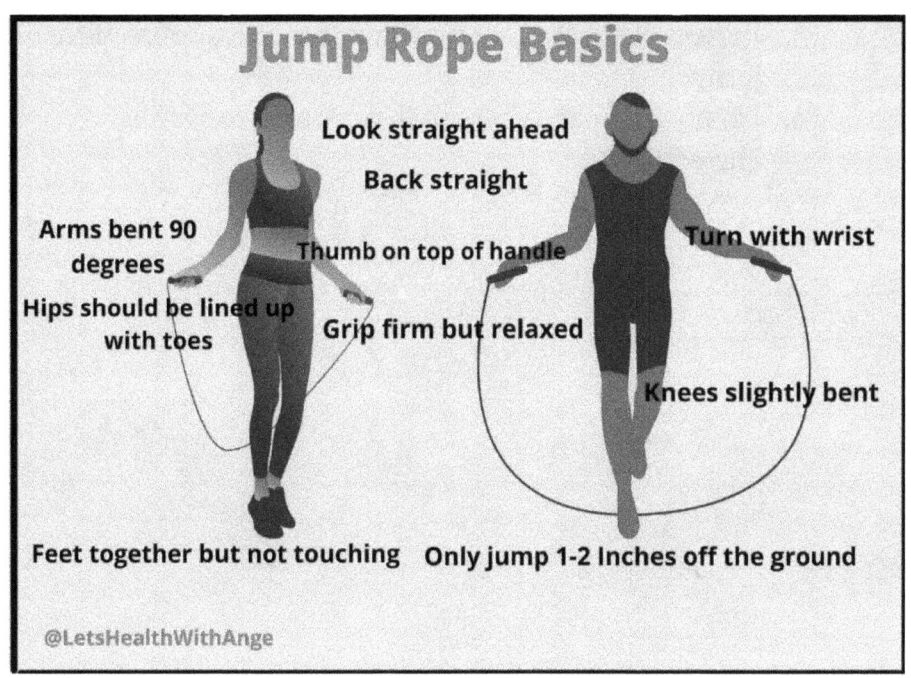

Jumping Tips

1. Holding the rope – Arms should be bent at 90 degrees and close to the body.
2. Grip handles loosely.
3. Swing rope with mostly wrist.
4. Control your arms and shoulders when swinging.
5. ONLY JUMP HIGH ENOUGH TO CLEAR THE ROPE.
6. Jump to a consistent tempo/rhythm.
7. Jump on the balls of your feet.
8. Keep your knees slightly bent while jumping.
9. Breathe.

Ways to improve with the jump rope:

1. Start slowly.
2. Challenge yourself to practice every day. One to two minutes a day can really show improvement in the long run.

3. Perfect the basics before moving on to more difficult jumps.
4. Do not compare yourself to anyone else's ability.
5. Have fun.

CHAPTER 4

ACCESSORIES

Buying a jump rope doesn't have to be complicated or expensive. In fact, you may already have a jump rope lying around at home. Use that to get started.

In "The Basics" chapter, I mentioned two types of basic jump ropes, but as with any fitness industry, there are more types of jump ropes and jump rope accessories available for different fitness purposes.

As you continue and advance in your jump roping and become a jump rope enthusiast, you may want to invest in the options.

Shopping for jump roping accessories can be exciting. You start thinking about the different types of jump ropes, how you can showcase your personality with different colors, different bag designs, cool jumping mats and things of this nature.

Below, I share some of the popular types of jump ropes and jump rope accessories:

Jump Ropes

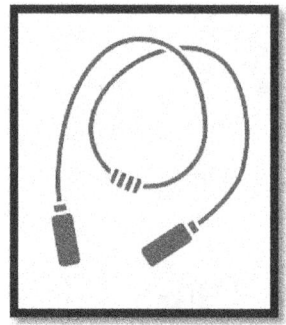

1. Speed Ropes – They are great for conditioning and are lightweight. Typically, speed ropes are very thin compared to other ropes.
2. Weighted Ropes – These ropes are just as the name implies; they are heavier in weight and tend to be thicker than speed ropes. The goal here is to work the upper body while jumping.
3. Outdoor Ropes – Usually, ropes made of PVC or nylon work best outdoors. But if you are not jumping on a mat, concrete will beat up any type of rope after consistent use.
4. Nylon Ropes – They are great for beginners. They usually have a slower turn rotation, which is great when learning different types of jumps.
5. Electric Ropes – These ropes usually have a counter feature on them. They keep count of your repetitions. These are convenient for jump rope challenges, or if you have a goal to do a lot of skips daily. They allow you to focus on jumping vs counting.

Jump Rope Mat

This accessory is important if you are jumping outside or at home. The main purpose of a jump rope mat is injury prevention. Concrete can be very unforgiving to the knees. If you are jumping on a gym floor or workout exercise room floor, you will not need a jump rope mat. Some mats are circular; others are rectangular. I personally prefer the circular ones. In addition to coming in different shapes, jump rope mats come in different thickness. You may be wondering if you can just use a yoga mat. No, you cannot. Yoga mats are not thick enough, and they are not shock absorbent.

Jump Rope Bags and Storage

How you store and transport your jump ropes will become increasingly important as you spend a lot of money on jump ropes. Also, depending on how many jump ropes you have, having a good quality jump rope bag is a great way to transport your jump ropes around with you. Some jump rope brands also sell their own brand of bags.

When you have more than one jump rope, you may want to invest in ways to maintain the longevity of your rope by purchasing a storage unit. Wall mounted hooks, carry bags, and standing jump rope racks are common ways to store jump ropes.

Sports Braces

This next accessory I will discuss is not as fun to shop for as some of the other accessories, but it is very important. If you are injured or have areas of your body that need a little bit more support, then you will need this next item. For example, sometimes you might hear someone say the reason they do not jump rope is because they have existing ankle problems or struggle with carpal tunnel in their wrist. These are reasons why people say that either they can't jump rope or why they stopped jumping rope. This may be your personal situation. Thanks to sports technology and rehabilitative technology, there are many different types of muscular supports available. Some excellent supports to invest in, if you have ailments, are knee braces, wrist support, compression sleeves (for knees, legs, shoulders, elbows, calves), back support, and ankle braces.

Chapter 5

The Jump Rope Tricks

I'm going to share a few different jump rope tricks with you, most will be used in the training workouts. You can add others to workouts that have a "freestyle" section, or you can add them to your daily freestyle jumping sessions to add variety.

Before I break them down, remember that jump rope tricks that can be done forward, in most cases, can also be done backwards. Another important note is that the terms "single jump" and "double jump" are not referring to a trick. Those terms refer to timing. Single jumps are when a person jumps once per turn of the rope; in other words, one turn one jump. Double jumps are two jumps per one turn of the rope; in other words, for every one turn of the rope, there will be one jump over rope and one jump between the next turn (and the next jump).

As you continue to dive into this handbook, you may be thinking to yourself, "Will this jump rope training program work for me? I barely know how to jump.," Or you may say to yourself, "I haven't jumped in years; I could never do the jumps or tricks I see others doing with a jump rope."

My advice is simple. Tell yourself to be quiet and just pick up the rope and start jumping. The bottom line is that the more you do something the better you will get. This is called practice.

In order to learn a jump rope trick and master it, YOU MUST PRACTICE. There is no "trick" to learning the tricks. (See what I did there. That was my attempt at a word play joke.) But seriously, you have to practice the jump rope tricks over and over again until you can confidently say, "I know that trick." Typically, performing a jump rope trick for 10 repetitions without messing up is proof that you have learned that trick.

I will divide the jump rope tricks into rounds. Round 1 is the, "I'm just starting to jump (beginner)" round. Round 2 is the, "I can jump pretty good (intermediate)" round. Round 3 is the, "I am ready for some challenges (advanced)" round.

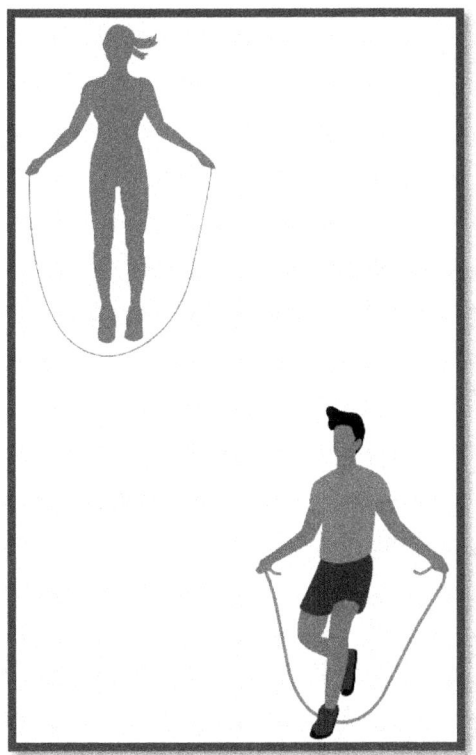

Here are the tricks that you will learn:

Round 1 Beginner Tricks

1. Basic Bounce

2. Side to Side (Skier)
3. Front to Back (Bell)
4. Jog Step
5. Side Jack (Side Straddle)
6. Playground Hop

Round 2 Intermediate Tricks

1. Boxer Shuffle
2. Arm Cross
3. Side Swing Jump
4. Side to Side Swing Jump
5. Front Jack (Front Straddle)
6. Rocking Chair
7. High Knee

Round 3 Advanced Tricks

1. Side Jack Cross
2. Double Under
3. 180 Degrees
4. 360 Degrees
5. Cross Jump
6. Cross Jog Step

Instructions:

Instructions are organized below. This will help you remember the steps and develop tempo.

- ➤ I use numbers to represent jumping tempo.
- ➤ The rhythm for the turn of rope is always 1, 2, 3, 4.
- ➤ The word "and" represents a jump or pause in between the main jump.

These concepts will make more sense to you as you go through each jump rope trick. Some people like to use a metronome or listen to music while jumping to help develop their tempo.

Round 1 Tricks

Jump Rope Tricks Tip: Try the movement without the rope, then grab your rope.

Basic Bounce

1. Rope starts behind you
2. Turn rope
3. Jump over

*Single – turn rope, jump over, repeat

- Jumping Tempo 1, 2, 3, 4

*Double – turn rope, jump over, jump, repeat

- Jumping Tempo 1 and, 2 and, 3 and, 4 and

Backwards Basic

1. Rope starts in front of you
2. Turn rope backwards
3. Jump over

*Single – turn rope, jump over, repeat

- Jumping Tempo 1, 2, 3, 4

*Double – turn rope, jump over, jump, repeat

- Jumping Tempo 1 and, 2 and, 3 and, 4 and

Side to Side (Skier)

1. Rope starts behind you
2. Turn rope
3. Jump to right side
4. Turn rope
5. Jump to left side

*Single – turn rope, jump over, repeat

- Jumping Tempo 1, 2, 3, 4

*Double – turn rope, jump over, jump, repeat

- Jumping Tempo 1 and, 2 and, 3 and, 4 and

Backwards Side to Side (Skier)

1. Rope starts in back
2. Turn rope
3. Jump to right
4. Turn rope
5. Jump to left side

*Single – turn rope, jump over, repeat

- Jumping Tempo 1, 2, 3, 4

*Double – turn rope, jump over, jump, repeat

- Jumping Tempo 1 and, 2 and, 3 and, 4 and

Front to Back (Bell)

1. Rope starts in back
2. Turn rope
3. Jump to front
4. Turn rope
5. Jump to back

*Single – turn rope, jump over, repeat

- Jumping Tempo 1, 2, 3, 4

*Double – turn rope, jump over, jump, repeat

- Jumping Tempo 1 and, 2 and, 3 and, 4 and

Backwards Front to Back (Bell)

1. Rope starts in front
2. Turn rope
3. Jump to front
4. Turn rope

5. Jump to back

*Single – turn rope, jump over, repeat

- Jumping Tempo 1, 2, 3, 4

*Double – turn rope, jump over, jump, repeat

- Jumping Tempo 1 and, 2 and, 3 and, 4 and

Single Hop

1. Starting stance – One leg down the other leg bet backwards
2. Turn rope
3. Jump over with just one foot
4. Repeat steps 2-3

*Single – turn rope, jump over, repeat

- Jumping Tempo 1, 2, 3, 4

*Double – turn rope, jump over, jump, repeat

- Jumping Tempo 1 and, 2 and, 3 and, 4 and

Jumps "2-6" can all be done as a single hop jump.

- Skier – both forwards and backwards
- Bell – both forwards and backwards

Jog Step

1. Jump rope starts behind you
2. Turn rope
3. When one jump off ground and jump off other foot over rope (jogging movement)
4. Turn rope
5. Foot off ground is now jumping foot, and waiting foot goes over rope (jogging movement)
6. Repeat

*Jumping Tempo 1, 2, 1, 2 (Left, Right, Left, Right)

Jog Step Backward

1. Jump rope starts in front of you
2. Turn rope
3. When one jump off ground and jump off other foot over rope (jogging movement)
4. Turn rope
5. Foot off ground is now jumping foot, and waiting foot goes over rope (jogging movement)
6. Repeat

*Jumping Tempo 1, 2, 1, 2 (Left, Right, Left, Right)

Side Jack (Side Straddle) Forward

1. Jump rope starts behind you
2. Basic bounce
3. Turn rope
4. Jump out (feet apart)
5. Turn rope
6. Jump in (feet together)
7. Repeat steps 3-6

*Jumping Tempo 1, 2, 1, 2 (feet together, feet apart, feet together, feet apart)

Side Jack (Side Straddle) Backward

1. Jump rope starts in front of you
2. Basic bounce
3. Turn rope backwards
4. Jump out (feet apart)
5. Turn rope backwards
6. Jump in (feet together)
7. Repeat steps 3-6

*Jumping Tempo 1, 2, 1, 2 (feet together, feet apart, feet together, feet apart)

High Knees

1. Jump rope starts behind you
2. Turn rope
3. Jump and bring up right knee, keep left leg down
4. Turn rope
5. Jump and bring up left knee, keep left leg down
6. Repeat steps 2-5

***Jumping Tempo 1, 2, 1, 2 (Left, Right, Left, Right)**

Round 2 Tricks

Jump Rope Tricks Tip: Start each trick with 4 basic jumps.

1. **One Foot Tap Boxer Shuffle**
   1. Jump, alternating your weight from right foot to left foot

*Jumping Tempo 1, 2, 1, 2 (left foot/lean, right foot/lean, left foot/lean, right foot/lean)**

2. **Double Foot Tap Boxer Shuffle**
   1. Jump alternating your weight from right foot to left foot
   2. Jump/tap foot twice before shifting weight to the other foot.

*Jumping Tempo 1-1, 2-2, 1-1, 2-2 (left foot/lean, left foot/lean, right foot/lean, left foot/lean, left foot/lean right foot/lean, right foot/lean)**

3. **Arm Cross Jump**
   1. Basic bounce
   2. Basic bounce
   3. Basic bounce
   4. Basic bounce
   5. Elbow to elbow as rope comes over your head
   6. Fist facing down
   7. Jump through the opening
   8. Turn wrist to swing rope back over head
   9. Open arms back up
   10. Repeat steps 5-9

*Can also be done with single hop jump**

4. **Side Swing**
   1. Start with hands close together holding jump rope – positioned in front of the stomach area
   2. Keep elbows bent at sides

3. Move both hands in a figure 8 motion – when turning to the right side, the left wrist will be on top of the right wrist
4. Continue to move both hands in a figure 8 motion – when turning to the left side, the right wrist will be on top of the left wrist

5. **Side Swing Jump**
   1. Start with hands close together holding jump rope – positioned in front of the stomach area
   2. Keep elbows bent at sides
   3. Move both hands in a figure 8 motion – when turning to the right side, the left wrist will be on top of the right wrist
   4. When turning to the left side, the right wrist will be on top of the left wrist
   5. As the rope moves from the side to the stomach open up the rope and jump through. Turning the rope over your head.

*Can also be done with single hop jump

6. **Front Straddle**
   1. Start with basic bounce
   2. Turn Rope
   3. Then jump with Right foot forward, Left foot backward
   4. Turn Rope
   5. Then jump left foot forward, right foot backward
   6. Repeat steps 3-5

7. **Rocking Chair**

In order to complete the rocking chair trick, I suggest you first master the front straddle trick.
   1. Start with rope behind you and feet spread like the front straddle (so either left foot forward, right foot back, or right foot forward, left foot back)
   2. Then as you turn the rope, jump/lean forward on your front foot

3. Turn rope, jump/lean backward on your back foot
4. Continue "rocking" back and forth between front leg and back leg while turning the rope.

8. **Playground Hop (Kick)**
    1. Jump rope starts behind you
    2. Basic Bounce (feet shoulder length apart)
    3. Turn Rope
    4. Jump and kick out right foot
    5. Turn rope
    6. Basic bounce (feet shoulder length apart)
    7. Turn Rope
    8. Jump and kick out left foot
    9. Repeat steps 2-8

*Jumping Tempo 1-1, 2-2, 1-1, 2-2

9. **Criss Cross Jump**
    1. Feet together
    2. Jump over rope
    3. Straddle apart
    4. Jump over rope
    5. Right leg in front (goes all the way left), left leg in back (goes all the way right)
    6. Jump over rope
    7. Straddle apart
    8. Left leg in front (goes all the way right), right leg in back (goes all the way left)
    9. Jump over rope
    10. Repeat 3-9

*Jumping Tempo 1, 2, 3, 4

Round 3 Tricks

Most round 3 tricks are just a combination of round 1 and round 2 tricks. For this reason, most of the round 3 jumps do not have instructions.

Jump Rope Tricks Tip: Learn the jump at a slow tempo. Wait until you can do it 10 times successfully before speeding up tempo.

1. **Double Unders (Dubs)**

The double under jump is 2 rope turns for 1 jump.
Double Unders require you to jump a little higher off the ground and land on the balls of your feet lightly. The best way to describe this is to imagine a penguin jumping. I know it sounds funny and you are thinking what?! But imagine a penguin jumping. That's the movement you need to master this trick.
   1. Rope starts behind us
   2. Basic Jump
   3. Basic Jump
   4. Basic Jump
   5. Basic Jump
   6. Turn rope double time – quick turn of wrist, keep arms around 90 degrees
   7. Jump on balls of feet
   8. Jump with toes pointing down

*Jump Rope Turn Tempo 1-1, 2-2, 3-3, 4-4
*Jump Rope Jump Tempo 1, 2, 3, 4

2. **180 Degrees Jump**
   1. Basic jump
   2. Basic jump
   3. Side swing
   4. Turn body backwards
   5. Backwards basic jump
   6. Backwards basic jump

3. **360 Degrees Jump**
   1. Basic jump
   2. Basic jump
   3. Side swing
   4. Turn body backwards
   5. Backwards basic jump
   6. Backwards basic jump
   7. High side swing
   8. Turn body forwards
   9. Basic jump
   10. Basic jump
4. **Arm Cross Jump**
   1. Basic bounce
   2. Basic bounce
   3. Basic bounce
   4. Basic bounce
   5. Elbow to elbow as rope comes over your head
   6. Fist facing down, arms close to body once rope is turned over the head
   7. Jump through the opening
   8. Turn wrist to swing rope back over head
   9. Keep elbow to elbow
   10. Jump through opening
   11. Repeat steps 8-10

*Can also be done with single hop jump

5. **Skier Arm Cross**
   a. Skier Jump combined with Arm Cross. This is a combination jump.
6. **Criss Cross Arm Cross**
   a. Criss Cross combined with Arm Cross. This is a combination jump.

Chapter 6

Time to Train

The workouts in the jump rope training plan are designed for you to use a jump rope and your body weight to achieve your goals.

Why do body weight exercises, calisthenics, combine well with jumping rope? First of all, calisthenics are very convenient. Between the jump rope and using your body weight for your workouts, the workouts are able to be done almost anywhere. Using these two exercise modalities allows for success by those who exercise often and those with little to no exercise experience. Another benefit of jump rope training and calisthenics is the fact that modifications can be made to help reduce the chance of injury and enjoy success.

The other important benefit of combining jumping rope and body weight exercises is time. No one wants to waste time and not get the results they were after. That's where this guide comes in and why it is so valuable! I've put in the time "getting it wrong", researching, and throughout that process, I figured out all the tricks to "get it right"!

I have also provided some "just in case" works. If you find yourself in the following situations, these additional workouts will be helpful.

1. Need to modify your workout plan and/or you need to rest from jumping rope and calisthenics due to injury or pain, I have included a walking workout training plan as well.
2. You have access to a gym, and would like to do additional workouts using gym equipment, I have included workouts that can be completed with gym equipment.

Now all you have to do with each workout is turn the page, and proven, result-getting, goal-attaining workouts are provided for you.

What do you need for your workouts?

1. Jump Rope
2. Stopwatch, Timer, or Something that will keep time for you (I use my smart watch and sometimes my phone)
3. Water
4. Exercise Mat (optional)
5. Dumbbells (optional)

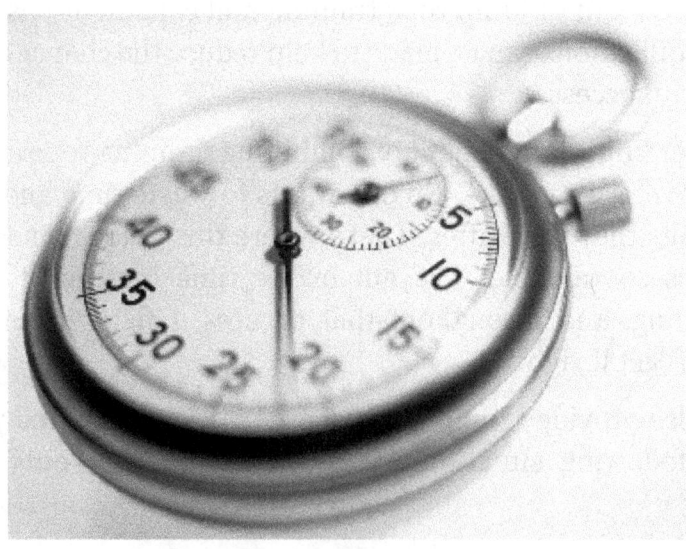

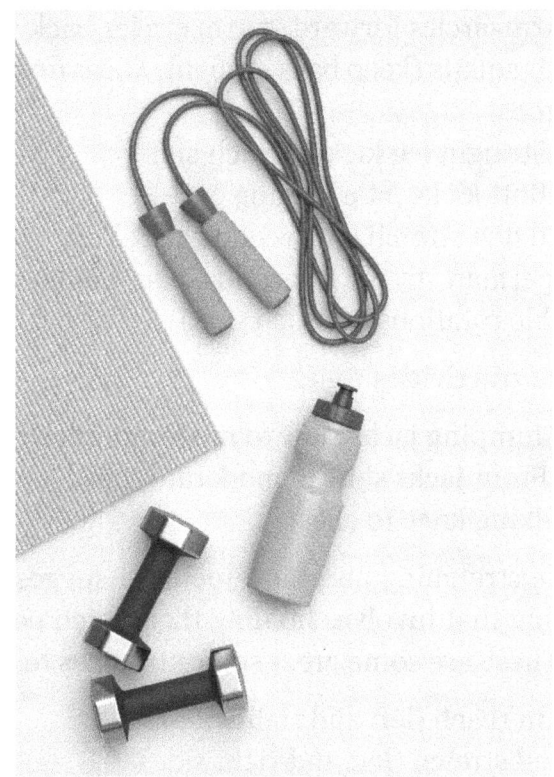

Warm- Up

Before diving into any workout, you have to first properly warm up. Take 5-10 minutes to prepare your body for your workout. Dynamic stretching is a great way to warm up your body. What is dynamic stretching? It is stretching through movement. Preferably, mimicking movements that you are about to engage in.

Here is a suggested warm-up before you begin any of the workouts:

1. March in place (be sure to simulate walking arm movements) 10 seconds
2. High knees in place (at a jogging pace) 10 seconds
3. 10 Calf raises (feet shoulder length apart) 10 repetitions
4. Slow jog in place 10 seconds
5. Lunge with twist (3 on each side)

6. 5 Arm circles forward, 5 arm circles backward
7. 5 Air squats (keep back straight, knees do not go in front of toes)
8. 10 Straight leg kicks (5 each side)
9. 10 Butt kicks (at a jogging pace)
10. Bird dog stretch (10 second each side)
11. Superman stretch 5 seconds, rest, then 5 more seconds
12. Ankle rotations (10 each side)

Repeat warm up activities #1-12

13. 10 Jumping jacks slow to moderate speed
14. 10 Front jacks slow to moderate speed
15. Walking knee to chest

After dynamic stretching and movements, I suggest doing some static stretching that involves holding the stretch position for 10-30 seconds. These are some great static stretches to engage in.

1. Sit in reach (left and right side)
2. Quad stretch (left and right side)
3. Lying hamstring stretch (left and right side)
4. Lower back stretch
5. Tricep stretch (left and right side)
6. Deltoid stretch (left and right side)

Cool Down

After each workout, be sure to cool down stretch. Take 5-10 minutes to engage in some static stretching of all major muscle groups. Spend extra time on any muscles that may be sore or that you focused on during the workout.

1. Sit in reach (left and right side)
2. Quad stretch (left and right side)
3. Lying hamstring stretch (left and right side)
4. Lower back stretch
5. Tricep stretch (left and right side)
6. Deltoid Stretch (left and right side)

Here is a sample beginner/intermediate workout schedule with <u>Daily Freestyle Sessions</u> included.

	Mon	Tues	Wed	Thurs	Fri	Sat	Sun
Week 1	Just Core Daily Freestyle Session	**Upper Body**	**Lower Body**	Rest Day	Daily Freestyle Session	Just Core	Rest Day
Week 2	**Full Body** Daily Freestyle Session	**Upper Body**	Just Core Daily Freestyle Session	**Just Jump**	Rest Day	Lower Body	**Rest Day**
Week 3	Just Core Just Jump	Rest Day	**Upper Body** Daily Freestyle Session	**Lower Body** **Just Core**	Daily Freestyle Session	**Full Body**	**Rest Day**
Week 4	Daily Freestyle Session	Just Core Daily Freestyle Session	**Lower Body**	**Rest Day**	Upper Body	**Full Body**	Daily Freestyle Session
Week 5	Daily Freestyle Session	**Rest Day**	Rest Day	**Upper Body**	Daily Freestyle Session	Just Core Daily Freestyle Session	**Just Jump**

I suggest you train three to five days per week.

- ➤ Three days if you are a beginner
- ➤ Four days if you are intermediate
- ➤ Five days advanced.

For each category—Just Core, Upper Body, Lower Body Fully Body, and Just Jump—there are a few choices of which workout you would like to complete on that training day.

Just Core and Just Jump are not full workouts, so they can be added to actual workout days or completed on rest days.

Each week strive to complete at least 1 Upper Body, 1 Lower Body, and 1 Full Body workout, as well as at least 1 Just Jump or 1 Just Core workout.

Each week you will complete 2-4 days of a set number of freestyle jumps, I will refer to these as "Daily Freestyle Session" repetitions.

Here is some fitness terminology that you need to know:

1. Repetitions—How many times you complete a jump. For example, 10 times jumping over the rope would equal 10 repetitions or reps.
2. A freestyle jump is when you jump using any jump rope trick you want.
3. Calisthenic—and exercise where body weight is used as the resistance

Below I have listed how many Daily Freestyle Session jumps you need to complete, or how long your session should be is based on your level.

Be sure to write these into your calendar.

Daily Freestyle Jump Session Chart

	Week 1	Week 2	Week 3	Week 4	Week 5
Beginner	50-100 Reps Or 1 Minutes	75-150 Reps Or 1:30 Minutes	100-200 Reps Or 2 Minutes	125-250 Reps Or 2:30 Minutes	150-300 Reps Or 3 Min
Intermediate	100-300 Reps Or 2 Minutes	150-250 Reps Or 2:30 Minutes	200-300 Reps Or 3 Minutes	250-350 Reps Or 3:30 Minutes	300-400 Reps Or 4 Minutes
Advanced	200-500 Reps Or 3-5:30 Minutes	250-350 Reps Or 3:30-6 Minutes	300-400 Reps Or 4-6:30 Minutes	350-450 Reps Or 4:30-7 Minutes	400-500 Reps Or 5-8 Minutes

Use the blank calendar provided to design a weekly schedule that works best for you.

I suggest you train 3-5 days per week. 3 days if you are beginner, 4 days intermediate, and 5 days advanced. Use the calendar template example I created above and add or subtract workouts as necessary.

Workout Schedule

	Mon	Tues	Wed	Thurs	Fri	Sat	Sun
Week 1							
Week 2							
Week 3							
Week 4							
Week 5							

Understanding Intensity and Target Heart Rate Zone

You will notice that for each exercise in the designed workouts, there is a recommended intensity level to perform that exercise. Intensity is how hard you are working (your heart). The way to assess your level of intensity is through monitoring your heart rate and comparing/using your target heart rate zone. Target Heart Rate Zone is a numerical range of heart beats per minute that represents the level of a person's intensity from low, moderate, to high intensity. Knowing your specific range and monitoring your heart rate during exercise allows you to safely exercise as well as determine intensity.

In order to use your target heart rate zone to determine your level of intensity effectively, you must first learn what your target heart rate zone is.

Here are the steps to calculating your target heart rate zone. If you are thinking, "No thanks, I don't have the time to calculate all this" or "No thanks, I hate math", there are online target heart rate zone calculators, and I will also share with you a general target heart rate zones chart that you can use.

Finding Your Target Heart Rate Zone

Step 1 Find your resting heart rate.

Ideally, this should be found first thing in the morning before you have consumed any food or got up and moving for the day. I will refer to the resting heart rate as RHR for the remainder of this section.

To find your heart rate you can use your wrist or neck. Do not use your thumb to count; use your middle and index finger. Count the number of beats for 60 seconds or count the number of beats for 6 seconds and multiply that number by 10.

My RHR = _____

Now that you have your resting heart rate, let's move on.

Step 2 Find your maximum heart rate.

It does require a little math, but you got this.

220 - Your Age = _____ Maximum Heart Rate (MHR)

My MHR = --------------- _____

Step 3 Find your target heart rate zone.

MHR____ - RHR _____ = _____ x .60 = _____ + RHR _____ = **Low Intensity**_____

MHR____ - RHR _____ = _____ x .70 = _____ + RHR _____ =**Moderate Intensity**_____

MHR____ - RHR _____ = _____ x .80 = _____ + RHR _____ = **High Intensity**_____

Low Intensity _____

Moderate Intensity_____

High Intensity_____

Here's an example:

Jamie is 40 years old. She has a maximum heart rate of 180 (MHR). She has a resting heart rate (RHR) of 60.

MHR <u>180</u> - RHR <u>60</u> = 120 x .60 = 72 + RHR 60 = **Low Intensity** 132

MHR <u>180</u> - RHR <u>60</u> = 120 x .70 = 84 + RHR 60 = **Moderate Intensity** 148

MHR <u>180</u> - RHR <u>60</u> = 120 x .80 = 96 + RHR 60 = **High Intensity** 156

Low Intensity 132

Moderate Intensity 148

High Intensity 156

*There's also websites and apps that can calculate your target heart rate zone for you.

Now that you have your numbers, let me explain how it works.

Once you start your workout, you will periodically check your intensity level during the workout by finding your heart rate (using neck, wrist, or a smart watch).

I suggest counting the number of beats for six seconds and then multiplying the number by 10. It saves time to do it this way, but for more accuracy, you can always count for 1 minute.

Once you have that number, you will "plug it in" or compare it to your target heart rate zone intensity levels. If you are below your low intensity number, you need to work a little harder to get your heart rate up. If you are higher than your high intensity level, then take a longer rest or stop working out altogether. That's it. Pretty simple right?

Now, this isn't the ultimate decision-making tool as it relates to safety. Always listen to your body and trust your instincts. If you feel you need to stop the workout, then stop it. Your health and safety are the number one priority.

As your cardiovascular endurance and overall conditioning improves, your target heart rate zone will also fluctuate. Typically, you will have to work harder to be in your zone, which means it will require a greater amount of intensity for you to get into the target heart rate zone. That's a good thing. That means you have improved your overall heart health. This is one of the many reasons why target heart rate zone is such a valuable tool to use to determine your level of intensity.

I have created a cheat chart below of some target heart rate zones to give a basic range. These numbers aren't as accurate as they would be if you did them using your resting heart rate. I did not use a resting heart rate for these calculations. Please keep that in mind.

Age	Low Intensity	Moderate Intensity	High Intensity
25	117	136	156
30	114	133	152
35	111	129	148
40	108	125	144
45	105	122	140
50	102	118	136
55	99	115	132
60	96	112	128
65	93	109	124

Now grab your jump rope, time to train!

CHAPTER 7

THE WORKOUTS

JUST CORE 1

Warm-Up and Stretch

Exercise	Duration/Reps	Intensity	Rest
Jumping Jacks	25	Moderate	10 seconds
Calf Raises	10	Moderate	
Basic Bounce	30 seconds to 1 minute	High	
High Knees	30 seconds to 1 minute	High	10 seconds
Russian Twist	30 seconds to 1 minute	Moderate	
Crunches	30 seconds	Moderate	30 seconds

Jog Step	30 Seconds	High	10 seconds
Plank Walk Out	30 seconds to 1 minute	High	10 seconds
Front Jacks	30 seconds	Low	10 seconds
Sit Ups with A Twist	30 seconds	Moderate	
Rest			30 seconds to 1 minute

Repeat x 3 Beginner OR for 5 Minutes

Repeat x 4 Intermediate OR for 7 Minutes

Repeat x 5 Advance OR for 15 Minutes

Cool Down and Stretch

JUST CORE 2

Warm-Up and Stretch

Exercise	Duration or Reps	Intensity	Rest
Plank	25 seconds	Low	10 seconds
Crunches	10	Low	
Mountain Climbers	10	Low	
Alternating Heel Taps	6	Low	10 seconds
Bicycle Crunches	10	Low	
Curl Ups	15	Low	10 seconds
Leg Lifts	10	Low	10 seconds
Russian Twist	6	Low	10 seconds
Rest			30 seconds to 1 minute

Repeat x 3 Beginner OR for 5 Minutes

Repeat x 4 Intermediate OR for 7 Minutes

Repeat x 5 Advance OR for 15 Minutes

Cool Down and Stretch

JUST CORE 2
Warm-Up and Stretch

Exercise	Duration/Repetitions	Intensity	Rest
Sit Ups	30 seconds	Moderate	
Russian Twist	20 seconds	Moderate	Rest 30 seconds
Leg Lifts	30 seconds	High	Rest 30 Sec
Bicycle Crunches	20 seconds	Moderate	Rest 30 seconds
Mountain Climbers	30 seconds	Moderate	Rest 30 seconds
Sit Ups with A Twist	20 seconds	Moderate	Rest 15 seconds
Plank	30 seconds	Low	
Windshield Wipers	15 seconds	Low	Rest 30 seconds
Plank Walk Out	45 seconds	Low	

Repeat x 3 Beginner OR for 5 Minutes

Rest			30 seconds to 1 minute

Repeat x 4 Intermediate OR for 7 Minutes

Repeat x 5 Advance OR for 15 Minutes

Cool Down and Stretch

FULL BODY 1
Warm-Up and Stretch

Exercise	Duration/Repetitions	Intensity	Rest
Jumping Jacks	30 seconds	Moderate	
Push Ups	30 seconds	Moderate	Rest 30 seconds
Basic Bounce	30 seconds	High	
Alternating Lunges	10 reps	Low	Rest 30 seconds
Side Straddle	30 seconds	Moderate	Rest 30 seconds
Standing Knee to Elbow (Right Side)	10 seconds	Moderate	
Bridge Arm Taps	20 reps	High	
Freestyle Jump	45 seconds	High	Rest 30 seconds
Plank Jacks	10 reps	Moderate	Rest 30 seconds

Squats	10 reps	Low	
Standing Knee to Elbow (Left Side)	10 Seconds	Moderate	
Rest			30 Seconds to 1 Minute

Repeat x 3 Beginner OR for 5 Minutes

Repeat x 4 Intermediate OR for 7 Minutes

Repeat x 5 Advance OR for 15 Minutes

Cool Down and Stretch

FULL BODY 2

Warm-Up and Stretch

Exercise	*Duration/Repetitions*	*Intensity*	*Rest*
Plank Walk Out	30 seconds	Moderate	
Pulse Squats	30 seconds	Low	Rest 30 seconds

Freestyle Jump	30 seconds	High	
Alternating Lunges	10 reps	Low	Rest 30 seconds
Side Straddle	30 seconds	Moderate	Rest 30 seconds
Sit Ups with a Twist	20 seconds	Moderate	
Plank Get Ups	10 reps	Moderate	Rest 30 seconds
Freestyle Jump	50 reps	High	Rest 30 seconds
Burpees	8 reps	Moderate	Rest 30 seconds
Squats	10 reps	Low	
Freestyle Jump	30 seconds	Moderate	
Rest			30 Seconds to 1 Minute
Repeat x 3 Beginner OR for 5 Minutes			

Repeat x 4 Intermediate OR for 7 Minutes

Repeat x 5 Advance OR for 15 Minutes

Cool Down and Stretch

FULL BODY 3

Warm-Up and Stretch

Exercise	Duration/Repetitions	Intensity	Rest
Basic Bounce Jump	30 seconds	High	15 seconds
Straddle Jump	30 seconds	Moderate	15 seconds
Plank Rotation	6	Moderate	
Skier Jump	30 seconds	High	10 seconds
Jog Step	30 seconds	Low	30 seconds
Alternating Lunges	6	Moderate	
Mountain Climbers	30 seconds	High	10 seconds
Plank Walk Out	30 seconds	High	10 seconds
Wide Leg Squats	6	Low	10 seconds

High Knee Jumps	30 seconds	
Rest		30 seconds to 1 minute
Repeat x 3 Beginner OR for 5 Minutes		
Repeat x 4 Intermediate OR for 7 Minutes		
Repeat x 5 Advance OR for 15 Minutes		
Cool Down and Stretch		

LOWER BODY 1

Warm-Up and Stretch

Exercise	Duration or Reps	Intensity	Rest
Freestyle Jump	30 seconds	Moderate	15 seconds
Wide Leg Squats	8	Low	
Toe Touches	30 seconds to 1 minute	High	
Alternating Squats (Wide and Regular)	8	Low	15 seconds
Quad Stretch	10 seconds per leg		
Alternating Lunges	8	Low	15 seconds
Wall Sits	15 seconds	Low	10 seconds
Knee to Feet	8	Moderate	10 seconds

Lying down hamstring Stretch	15 seconds per leg		
Pulsating Squats	8	Low	10 seconds
Rest			30 seconds to 1 minute
Repeat x 3 Beginner OR for 5 Minutes			
Repeat x 4 Intermediate OR for 7 Minutes			
Repeat x 5 Advance OR for 15 Minutes			
Cool Down and Stretch			

LOWER BODY 2

Warm-Up and Stretch

Exercise	Duration or Reps	Intensity	Rest
Boxer Shuffle	30 seconds	Moderate	10 seconds

Exercise	Reps	Intensity	Hold
Squat Front Kick	10	Moderate	
Side Leg Raises	8	High	
Squats hold Calf Raise	8	Moderate	10 seconds
Freestyle Jump	30 seconds	Moderate	
Alternating Lunges	8	Low	
Quad Stretch	15 seconds per leg		
Laying Hamstring Stretch	15 seconds per leg		
Laying Glute Flex Thrust	8	Moderate	10 seconds
Side Lunges	8	Low	10 seconds
Donkey Kicks	8	Moderate	
Rest			30 seconds to 1 minute

Repeat x 3 Beginner OR for 5 Minutes

Repeat x 4 Intermediate OR for 7 Minutes

Repeat x 5 Advance OR for 15 Minutes

Cool Down and Stretch

UPPER BODY 1

Warm-Up and Stretch

Exercise	Duration or Reps	Intensity	Rest
Jumping Jacks	45 seconds	Moderate	10 seconds
Plank Shoulder Taps	5	Low	
Basic Bounce	30 seconds to 1 minute	High	
Bear Crawls (Forwards and Backwards)	30 seconds to 1 minute	Moderate	10 seconds
Side to Side Jump	30 seconds to 1 minute	Moderate	
Chair Dips	10	Low	

Exercise	Duration	Intensity	Rest
Jog Step	30 seconds to 1 minute	High	10 seconds
Get Ups	30 seconds	Low	10 seconds
Freestyle Jump	45 seconds	Moderate	10 seconds
Close Arm Pushups	8	Low	
Rest			30 seconds to 1 minute

Repeat x 3 Beginner OR for 5 Minutes

Repeat x 4 Intermediate OR for 7 Minutes

Repeat x 5 Advance OR for 15 Minutes

Cool Down and Stretch

UPPER BODY 2

Warm-Up and Stretch

Exercise	*Duration or Reps*	*Intensity*	*Rest*
Boxer Shuffle	45 seconds	Moderate	10 seconds
Diamond Push ups	5	Low	
Plank	10	Low	
Freestyle Jump	30 seconds to 1 minute	High	
Plank Walk Outs	30 seconds to 1 minute	Low	10 seconds
Side Straddle Jump	30 seconds to 1 minute	Moderate	
Wide Arm Push Ups	5	Low	
Plank Jacks	30 Seconds to 1 minute	Moderate	10 seconds
Plank	45 seconds	Low	10 seconds
Pushups	8	Low	

Rest		30 seconds to 1 minute

Repeat x 3 Beginner OR for 5 Minutes

Repeat x 4 Intermediate OR for 7 Minutes

Repeat x 5 Advance OR for 15 Minutes

Cool Down and Stretch

JUST JUMP 1

Warm Up and Stretch

Exercise	Duration or Reps	Intensity	Rest
Jumping Jacks	15 seconds	moderate	10 seconds
Front Straddle	30 seconds	moderate	10 seconds
Basic Bounce	30 seconds to 1 minute	moderate	10 seconds
Jog Step	30 seconds to 1 minute	moderate	10 seconds
Basic Bounce	30 seconds to 1 minute	moderate	10 seconds
Side straddle	30 seconds to 1 minute	moderate	10 seconds
Basic Bounce	30 seconds to 1 minute	moderate	10 seconds
Freestyle Jump	30 seconds to 1 minute	moderate	10 seconds
Front Jumping Jacks	15 seconds	moderate	

Rest			30 seconds to 1 minute

Repeat x 3 Beginner OR for 5 Minutes

Repeat x 4 Intermediate OR for 7 Minutes

Repeat x 5 Advance OR for 15 Minutes

Cool Down and Stretch

JUST JUMP 1

Warm Up and Stretch

Exercise	Duration or Reps	Intensity	Rest
Boxer Shuffle	15 seconds	Moderate	10 seconds
Left Foot bounce	30 seconds	Moderate	10 seconds
Basic Bounce	30 seconds to 1 minute	High	30 seconds

Arm cross	30 seconds to 1 minute	Moderate	10 seconds
High knees	30 seconds to 1 minute	High	30 seconds
Criss cross feet	30 seconds to 1 minute	Moderate	10 seconds
Basic Bounce	30 Seconds to 1 minute	Moderate	10 seconds
Freestyle Jump	30 seconds to 1 minute	High	10 seconds
Right Foot	15 seconds	Moderate	
Rest			30 seconds to 1 minute

Repeat x 3 Beginner OR for 5 Minutes

Repeat x 4 Intermediate OR for 7 Minutes

Repeat x 5 Advance OR for 15 Minutes

Cool Down and Stretch

JUST JUMP 2
Warm Up and Stretch

Exercise	Duration or Reps	Intensity	Rest
Freestyle Jump	15 seconds	moderate	10 seconds
Backwards basic	30 seconds	moderate	10 seconds
Arm cross, side swing, jump, side swing	30 seconds to 1 minute	moderate	10 seconds
Arm cross	30 seconds to 1 minute	moderate	10 seconds
Jog Step	30 seconds to 1 minute	moderate	10 seconds
Kick Jumps	30 seconds to 1 minute	moderate	10 seconds
Basic Bounce	30 seconds to 1 minute	moderate	10 seconds
Freestyle Jump	30 seconds to 1 minute	moderate	10 seconds
Double Unders	15 seconds	moderate	

Rest		30 seconds to 1 minute
Repeat x 3 Beginner OR for 5 Minutes		
Repeat x 4 Intermediate OR for 7 Minutes		
Repeat x 5 Advance OR for 15 Minutes		
Cool Down and Stretch		

Extra Workout Tips

Depending on your fitness level, feel free to combine these jump rope focused workouts with a strength-training program.

When it comes to the jump rope tricks, if you do not know how to do one that is written in the workout, **MODIFY AS NECESSARY**. In other words, do a jump rope trick you can do.

I hope you have enjoyed the workouts. You are now one jump closer to reaching your health and fitness goals. Throughout your journey, remember that you are in competition with no one. Just continue to be patient and consistent, and you will accomplish your goals!

Chapter 8

The Acceleration Process

I know this is a book about jumping rope, but the acceleration tips I am about to share with you are not jump rope related. All of these tips are ways to potential accelerate your goal achievement process:

1. Intermittent fasting
2. Health apps
3. Goal setting
4. Habits
5. Nutrition
6. Water
7. Sleep
8. Energy

Intermittent Fasting

Intermittent fasting, or IF for short, is a fasting technique in which a person abstains from taking in or eating calories, and when a person takes in or consumes anything with calories. The most popular intermittent fasting schedule is known as 16:8. This is broken down into a 16 hour fasting window and an 8-hour eating window.

Why am I talking about intermittent fasting in a jump rope book? Well, combining IF with the jump rope training plan may accelerate your fitness and health goals. Here's why. Intermittent fasting forces the body to use stored energy (carbs), and once it burns through the stored energy, it then can use stored fat for energy, thus leading to more fat burning.

Other IF benefits besides fat burning may include improving insulin resistance, reducing inflammation in the body, and heart health.

Health Apps

Apps or applications for your phone or tablet can be a game changer. There are some helpful free apps that can not only assist with workouts, but also keep track of how many hours you have been intermittent fasting. They also provide information about what's happening during the fasting process.

1. Zero: Fasting and Health Tracker
2. Fastic: Fasting App

These next few apps will help you keep track of the time intervals during your workouts. They are all user friendly and have other features associated with them. They are available on both Apple and Android platforms.

1. Tabata HITT: Interval Timer
2. Tabata Timer: Interval Timer
3. SmartWOD Timer: WOD Timer

Goal Setting

The next acceleration tip is goal setting. Goals can be organized by the well-known SMART method. SMART is an acronym for: specific, measurable, attainable, realistic, and time bound. Once the goal has been organized using these "ingredients", it's time to write down the plan. The plan should include a section for your nutrition as well as a section for your fitness.

Here's an example: **Overall Goal** = Lose weight

| **Specific** | I would like to lose 15 pounds in 30 days. |

Measurable	I will weigh myself every 5 days for 30 days to see if I have lost 15 pounds.
Attainable	I have lost 2-4 pounds per week before, so I know losing 2 pounds per week for one month is possible for me.
Relevant	I would like to be healthier, and I am currently overweight. Losing 15 pounds will put me in the healthy weight category.
Time Bound	I would like to achieve this goal in 30 days.

My Plan
In order to lose at least 2 pounds per week, I will change my nutrition to mostly plant based, eat at a calorie deficit, and work out weekly. **Nutrition Plan:** Consume 6 to 8 cups of dark leafy greens every day. Drink at least ½ gallon of water every day. **Fitness Plan** = Work out 3 to 5 days per week.

Use the table below to organize your health/fitness related goal

Overall Goal =

_____

_____

Specific	
Measurable	
Attainable	
Realistic	
Time bound	

My Plan

Habits

A quick lesson on how to reprogram bad habits into great habits, and how to establish new beneficial habits; this is so critical to the success of your day to day fitness and health goals.

According to many experts, habits are generally formed and carried out in a series of steps. When I think of habit-forming, this is usually the sequence that occurs.

1. Some type of cue will trigger a habit response.
2. That response will either lead to a positive or negative reaction (habit), and consequence.
3. Whether it be a positive or negative reaction (habit), the habit response that is chosen tends to yield a rewarding feeling.

In my experience, often times if it is a negative response (habit), the rewarding or satisfying feeling will only be temporary and is usually followed by regret. Whereas, the positive response (habit), may not feel super satisfying at first, but it will not be followed by the feeling of regret, which in return is a rewarding feeling.

So how do we establish or improve current habits? Here are the three steps:

1. Recognize the cue (a cue is a signal).
2. Some examples of cues could be stress, feeling happy, feeling sad, feeling angry, or even an upcoming celebration or outing.
3. Decide what the response to that cue will be.

Follow through with a positive reaction (habit).

That's it! Now the challenge is to consistently choose the right habit. My advice: "Stay positive and give yourself some grace from time to time."

Nutrition

There's an old saying that when it comes to health and body composition, the process is 20% fitness and 80% nutrition. I agree with this saying.

With that being said, tighten up on your nutrition if you aren't already dialed in. Stick to as much whole foods and plant foods as possible. Eating plenty of dark leafy greens, low fat sources of protein, and daily consumption of fruit and vegetables is a good place to start. If you aren't reaching your goals in a timely manner, the first place I would investigate would be your nutrition.

Water

Water, water, and more water. Water makes up more than 70% of our body. It makes everything flow. Water can also aide in preventing dehydration. When it comes to increasing the amount of physical activity, bear in mind that it is important to drink water throughout the day and in the hours leading up to your workout.

A good rule of thumb is to drink half your weight in ounces each day. For instance, a 200-pound person would need to drink about 100 ounces of water per day.

Sleep

Strive to get 6-9 hours of sleep per night. Rest when you get opportunities. In order to recover properly, the body needs rest.

Energy

What about energy to train? Caffeine is usually the go to for most people. When consumed for energy to train, people often turn to pre-work supplements. Pre-workout supplements come in powder form, pre-mixed drinks, and pills. They are usually taken 15-20 minutes before a workout, and in addition to having caffeine, many have other ingredients that provide fitness-related benefits.

There are plenty of supplements that provide energy on the market; I would be here all day listing them. But in general, you have:

1. Caffeine pills
2. Coffee
3. Pre-workout mixes and drinks
4. Herbal teas (that contain caffeine)

Quick boss tip about caffeine: cycle on and off of it, and only use it when you absolutely need it.

CHAPTER 9

NO PAIN, NO SETBACKS

If you have ever experienced an injury, you already know the importance of being proactive against injury or getting reinjured. With that being said, try to contain your excitement to jump right into the training schedule and really take in what I am about to share with you.

You should not jump when you are hurt. Being sore from exercise and being in actual pain are different. Recognize the difference and act accordingly.

Now that we have established that, I want to share with you some suggestions to help avoid injury.

First things first: be sure to stay properly hydrated. I already went into more detail about the importance of water in the acceleration process, Chapter 8. But the bottom line is that when it comes to water, just drink it. Drink plenty of it and drink it throughout the day.

The next big topic when it comes to injury prevention and recovery is warming up. The importance of properly warming up can't be stressed enough. Injury prevention starts with preparing your body for the more intense exercises to come. You should spend 3-10 minutes at least warming up before you stretch (and work out).

One of my favorite analogies to share with my physical education students when discussing the importance of warming up is the "frozen chicken" analogy. Now, I did not come up with this idea; I borrowed it from a coworker, added a bit of my personality to it, and based on how well students understand the concept as a result of it, I kept using it.

So here goes it: "Imagine you are a frozen chicken and someone bought you from the grocery store and stored you in the freezer until it was time for you to stretch and work out. As soon as they take you out of the freezer, they start bending you around (stretching you). What do you think is going to happen? You are probably thinking right now, "I (being the chicken) will snap or break." That's exactly it! So, what makes more sense to do before bending and stretching the frozen chicken? Hopefully, you are thinking, *Thaw it out or warm it up,* as that is the correct response!

So, that explains the analogy. And just like that frozen chicken, your muscles need to warm up as well to prevent them from being injured (or snapping).

So, long story short, make sure you warm up properly. I've given a great warmup protocol that includes dynamic movements, but feel free to modify it or add other exercises as necessary to fit your personal needs.

Now that you have nailed the warm up, let's talk about the next tip in injury prevention, and that is the cool down.

This is often left out of the workout, because after someone has just busted their tail working out, most just want to relax, leave the gym, or are just not in the mood to stretch and cool down. This usually leads to people skipping the cool down.

Sound about right? Well they/you are not alone. However, a proper cool down (and static stretch) session can be great for injury prevention and lessening muscle soreness.

Next up is to wear and use quality equipment, braces, and accessories. All of the aforementioned tips will be useless if the equipment you are using is dangerous. Make sure you are using athletic shoes with shock absorption and good soles. If you are jumping outside, be sure to jump with a mat. Lastly, if you have previous injuries, wear the proper braces or support while jumping.

When it comes to jumping correctly (proper jumping form) to avoid injury, remember that practice makes perfect.

Having good jumping technique will help prevent injury or reinjury. Jumping technique is especially critical when it comes to how high you jump off the ground and how much you bend your knees. Remember that your knees should only bend slightly. You do not want to put unnecessary stress and strain on your joints and major muscles. And you should only jump high enough to clear the rope, which is about 1-2 inches of the ground.

If you do get hurt or are already injured, utilize the R.I.C.E. technique to help recover. The acronym RICE stands for Rest, Ice, Compression, and Elevation. So, whatever body part or muscle is ailing, the first order of business is to see a physician to determine the severity of the situation, then rest it, ice it, compress the area (with a bandage or a brace), and keep it elevated as much as possible.

Chapter 10

"Just In Case"

This chapter is geared for the "just in case scenarios". The first just in case scenario is if you get injury, or are unusually sore. The second just in case scenario is for those of you how have gym memberships and can handle a gym workout plan in addition to your jump rope workout plans.

Injury

Unfortunately, setbacks sometimes happen, even when we jump correctly and utilize the proper equipment/accessories. If you find yourself in a situation where you are unable to jump rope (for whatever reason), this is your, "JUST IN CASE" plan walking workout plan. Why is walking a great alternative? For starters, walking is a great form of cardiovascular endurance. Activities that improve our cardiovascular endurance are great for strengthening the heart. Cardiovascular endurance activities are also great for the lungs.

What I enjoy about walking is it is low impact activity. Therefore, if you are experiencing soreness or even recovering from an injury, you can still walk (in most cases). Walking also strengthens the leg muscles, improves mood, improves balance, and engages core muscles.

The next page details a warm up that's great for preparing to do your walking workout. It is both low intensity and low impact.

Feel free as you go through the workout to add other stretches (that you can physically handle) as necessary.

JUST IN CASE – Walking Plan

Warm Up

EXERCISE	DURATION/REPS	INTENSITY
Calf Raises	10	Moderate
March In Place	10	Moderate
Donkey Kick Backs	10	Moderate
Marching High Knees	10	Moderate

Let's Walk Treadmill Plan

	DURATION/REPS	INTENSITY	SPEED
Walk	5 Minutes	Low	0 Incline
Stretch (Lower and Upper Body)	As Needed	Low	
Walk	15 Minutes	Moderate	0-2 Incline (if soreness and/or injury and ability allows) 2.5-2.8 mph
Walk	15 Minutes	Moderate	Increase Incline by 1-2 (if soreness and/or injury or

			ability allows) 2.5-3.2 mph
Walk	5 Minutes	Low	Decrease Incline to 0 2.0-2.8 mph

*if you are walking outside, pace yourself by your intensity level.

Gym Access

If you have a gym membership and feel you can physically handle a gym workout in addition to your jump rope workout plan, then this "just in case" gym plan is for you to use.

- Workouts are designed to use basic gym equipment such as dumbbells, bench, and cable machines. There are some exercises that utilize a smith machine, but I provide 2 options if your gym does not have one of those have options.
- You will use the same warm-up protocol as the one used for your jump rope workouts or if you do your jump rope workout first, you should already be "warmed up" to complete these exercises.

Gym Workouts – Lower Body Focus

Lower Body

	Major Muscles	*Duration/Reps*	*Intensity*
Complete Warm Up		5 Minutes	Low
Stretch		As Needed	Low
(Dumbbell) Squats			Moderate
(Dumbbell) Lunges			Moderate
Reverse Lunges			Moderate
Dead Lift			
Leg Extension			
Leg Curls			

Hip Thrust

Guidelines

- ➤ For all exercises use the following method of choosing how much weight to use:
  - Heavy Weight -3 to 5 Reps
  - Moderate Weight – 8 to 12 Reps
  - Low Weight – 10-15 Reps

- ➤ Since you are adding these workouts to an existing workout plan only choose:
  - 3 to 5 exercises to complete each workout (Beginner)
  - 5 to 7 exercises to complete each workout (Intermediate and Advanced)

Gym Workout
Gym Workout – Upper Body Focus

Upper Body - Pull

	DURATION/REPS	INTENSITY
Complete Warm Up	5 Minutes	Low
Stretch	As Needed	
Lat Pull Down (Latissimus Dorsi)	8-12	Moderate
Deadlift	10-15	Low
Face Pulls (Back)	8-12	Moderate
Bicep Curl (Biceps)	8-12	Moderate
Bent Over Barbell Row (Back)	8-12	Low
Single Dumbbell Row (Back)	8-12	Heavy
Overhead Tricep Extension (Tricep)	8-12	Moderate

Hammer Curl (Bicep)	8-12	Moderate

For all exercises use the following method of choosing how much weight to use:

- Heavy Weight-3 to 5 Reps
- Moderate Weight – 8 to 12 Reps
- Low Weight – 10-15 reps

Upper Body - Push

	Duration/Reps	*Intensity*
Complete Warm Up	5 Minutes	Low
Stretch	As Needed	
Bench Press	8-12	Moderate
Dumbbell Shoulder Press	8-12	Moderate
Arnold Press	8-12	Moderate

For all exercises use the following method of choosing how much weight to use:

- Heavy Weight-3 to 5 Reps
- Moderate Weight – 8 to 12 Reps

Let's Stay Connected

Thanks for reading this handbook. I hope it exceeded your expectations. You are now ready to jump like a boss! Now go out there and reach those fitness goals.

Be sure to keep in contact with me. I'd love to hear about your successes and experiences along your journey.

- Email letshealth@yahoo.com
- Instagram @ LetsHealthWithAnge
- Books and guides available on Amazon
- Sea Moss/Bladderwrack Liquid Drops (Strawberry) available at https://letshealth.biz

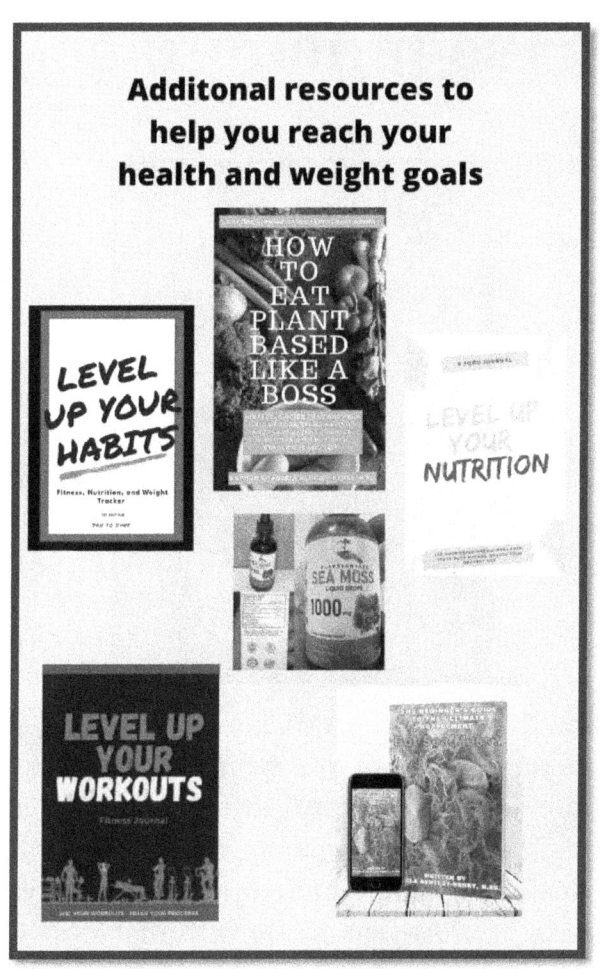

ABOUT THE AUTHOR

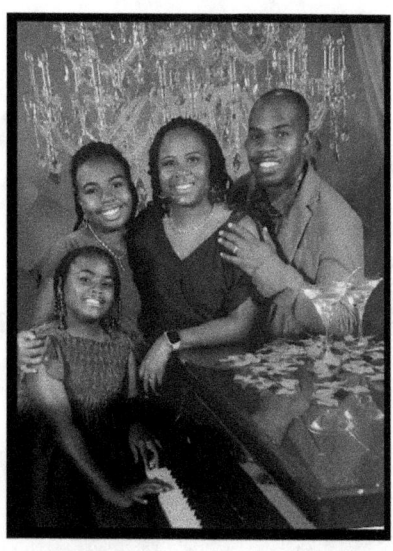

Educating and inspiring others to live a healthy and fit lifestyle is Angela's passion. Seeing others benefit from plant-dominated nutrition combined with physical activity, such as jumping rope and body weight exercise, is a personal mission she has taken on since the death of her grandmother. Angela watched her grandmother fight a 20-year battle with diabetes (which led to strokes, feeding tubes, being wheelchair bound, and the need for a pacemaker). Before her grandmother's death, Angela did not know there was a way to battle diabetes, hypertension, and other lifestyle diseases. She now believes in the power of plants and regular fitness activity. Her life has been proof.

Angela was very active throughout her childhood and teenage years. Angela played sports in school and was a standout basketball player. After college, she played semiprofessional basketball. Because of her active lifestyle, Angela appeared to be very healthy. She did not have any body weight issues, and thus saw no reason to change the way she ate (which was not whole food or plant-dominated). However, over time, those unhealthy eating habits caught up with her. In 2015 (the same year her grandmother passed away), Angela was diagnosed with pre-diabetes and was severely overweight. Jumping rope, regular fitness, and plant-based eating is the reason why Angela has lost over 50 pounds and reversed her pre-diabetes, and is now living a healthier, higher quality life.

Angela believes that plants provide her with the fuel she needs to engage in activities she loves, like playing basketball, staying busy with her daughters, jumping rope, and working out. Angela hopes to inspire others to pick up a jump rope and eat plants with her story.

Education:
- Master of Science in Education – Nova Southeastern University
- Bachelor of Science – University of Central Florida

Certifications:
- Plant Based Cooking – Rouxbe, Forks Over Knives
- Health Education – Florida Department of Education
- Physical Education – Florida Department of Education
- Certified Fitness Trainer – International Sports Science Association
- Weight Management Specialist – The National Council for Certified Personal Trainers
- Punk Rope Jump Rope Instructor – Punk Rope, Inc.

Professional:
- Author
- CEO of LETS Health
- Physical Education and Health Teacher
- Track, Soccer, Basketball Coach

SPECIAL THANKS

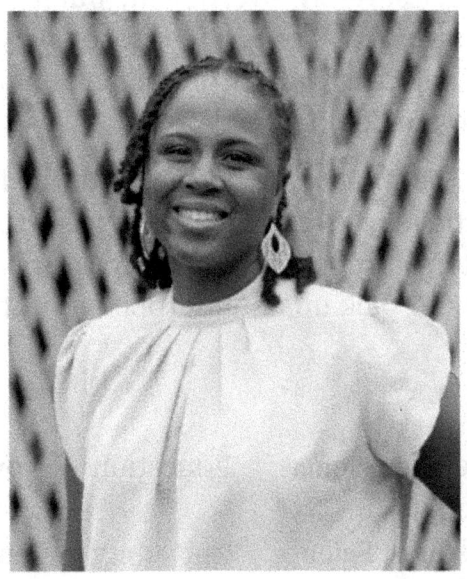

First, I would like to say THANK GOD for his never-ending and often undeserved blessings (His Grace and Mercy).

To my loving husband, Chris: Thank you for your unending support of all my aspirations. I love you, babes.

To my daughters, Abriana and Aleah: Always remember that the sky is the limit. Continue to believe in yourselves and go after what you want in life. Thanks for always making Mommy feel like she can do anything.

To my mom, Elzora: Thank you for consistently making me feel as though I have superpowers and can accomplish anything! Whenever I'm in need, you come through. You have always been and will forever be my role model.

To my siblings: Thank you for always speaking excellence over me. I appreciate it.

To my family and friends (you know who you are): Thank you for your support. I know I'm a little outside the box, but you love me anyway.

To my Sister-in-Love, Chrystal Campbell: thank you for your smile, the way you loved on your nieces, and your ability to always "be present". Rest in heaven.

Last but not least, this guide and my desire to help and inspire others to reach their fitness and health goals are dedicated to my loving grandmother, Atlee Fletcher Grady. Continue to rest in peace. I miss you. Love, Angie.

REFERENCE

Baker J.A. (1968). Comparison of Rope Skipping and Jogging as Methods of Improving Cardiovascular Efficiency of College Men. Research Quarterly. American Association for Health, Physical Education and Recreation, Vol. 39(2).

https://www.tandfonline.com/doi/abs/10.1080/10671188.1968.10618043

www.ingramcontent.com/pod-product-compliance
Lightning Source LLC
Chambersburg PA
CBHW070538030426
42337CB00016B/2255